Grapefruit
Seed
EXTRACT

POWERFUL PROTECTION AGAINST
VIRUSES, BACTERIA, FUNGI AND
OTHER HARMFUL MICROBES

Louise Tenney, M.H.

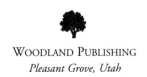

WOODLAND PUBLISHING
Pleasant Grove, Utah

© 2000
Woodland Publishing
P.O. Box 160
Pleasant Grove, UT
84062

ISBN 1-58054-081-3

Table of Contents

Introduction

IN A WORLD WHERE DRUGS ARE BECOMING INCREASINGLY ineffective for many types of parasites, the benefits of natural supplements are becoming more important. Scientists and researchers from many countries are developing more interest in herbs and natural products, and more and more doctors are validating the use of such supplements for many problems as daily discoveries make it into the news and reputable scientific journals.

One such natural alternative is grapefruit seed extract (GSE). GSE is a powerful, broad-spectrum antimicrobial that is being used to fight many types of bacteria, viruses, protozoa, fungi and other microbes. It can be used topically and internally without side effects and has not only been tested and approved by the FDA, USDA and the Pasteur Institute in France, but also has been supported by physicians in dozens of cities in the United States, as well as abroad.

Scientific laboratories and universities both in America and abroad have been uncovering the properties of grapefruit seed since the seventies, and gradually this extract has made its way into hospitals and households all over the United States. In fact, GSE may one day replace current antibiotics and toxic disinfectants. What exactly makes GSE better than more traditional antimicrobials?

THE ADVANTAGES OF GSE

1. GSE IS A BROAD SPECTRUM ANTIMICROBIAL. This means that it has the ability to fight a number of different types of bacteria, viruses, fungi and other microbes. This ability is especially important, because often we are not sure of the exact invader or combination of invaders that are attacking the body.

2. GSE IS VERY POWERFUL AND EFFECTIVE, even when greatly diluted. In fact, in a recent study at the Bio Research Laboratories of Redmond, Washington, GSE was compared to iodine, chlorox bleach, tea tree oil and colloidal silver in order to determine which substance worked best against certain microbes. GSE came out on top against all five microbes tested—*Candida albicans, Staphylococcus aureus, Salmonella typhi, Streptococcus faecium and E. coli.* GSE's ability was by far the best, even when using only moderate levels, compared to higher levels used with the bleach and colloidal silver. Researchers determined that GSE is ten to one hundred times more effective than chlorine and ten times more effective than colloidal silver on these organisms. In fact, GSE proved effective down to 10 ppm, or 1/100,000 dilution.

3. GSE IS NONTOXIC TO ANIMALS AND HUMANS—even pregnant women and children. GSE has been used at several times the recommended amount without reported side effects. A report from Northview Pacific Laboratory stated that even though a person would most likely not consume more than 1,000 mg a day, a person weighing 132 pounds could safely consume 300,000 mg a day—or 5,000 mg per kg of their body weight.

4. GSE POSES VERY LITTLE THREAT TO THE BENEFICIAL BACTERIA (i.e. Lactobacillus and Bifidobacterium) in the intestines and urogenital tract. Unlike prescription antibiotics, GSE does not upset the natural flora balance which could lead to candida infection. In fact, GSE may actually encourage the growth of good bacteria by inhibiting the microbes that are competing for its space and food.

5. GSE IS WELL-RESEARCHED. More than eighty scientific laboratories and forty universities have researched GSE in hundreds of studies

to check its toxicity and properties. And more research continues to be done on safe usage and its broad range of applications.

6. GSE IS BIODEGRADABLE, according to reports in 1994 from Bio Research Laboratories. Because of its organic nature, say researchers, it is completely safe for the environment and may be useful to replace pesticides.

7. GSE IS A PRODUCT OF NATURAL PLANT SOURCES—namely the seeds, pulp and white membranes, unlike some commercial antibiotics which may be derived from petroleum or coal tar.

8. UNLIKE MANY COMMERCIAL PRESCRIPTION DRUGS, GSE rarely causes allergic reactions, especially those as severe as anaphylactic shock—even if taken on a regular basis. If you have allergies to citrus, try a patch test first, and remember that GSE is acidic and can irritate the stomach and intestinal lining if taken in high dosages. It can also irritate the skin if used undiluted.

9. GSE IS MORE AFFORDABLE THAN MOST OTHER SUBSTANCES used for the same purposes. The average treatment costs about fifty to seventy-five cents a day, and it is derived from an inexpensive source (grapefruit seeds and pulp). In addition, it is used in such small amounts, that even a small bottle of concentrate can last quite a while. GSE also has no real expiration date—as long as it is not tampered with or kept at extreme temperatures, it can last for quite some time.

10. GSE IS VERY COMPATIBLE WITH OTHER TREATMENTS and can be mixed with vegetable oils, alcohol, water, shampoos, lotions and other substances for topical use, and with water, juices and syrups for internal use. It can even be mixed into pet food for sick animals. And not only are herbal combinations sometimes more effective than single herb treatments, they are also likely to be better preserved when mixed with GSE. Tea tree oil, echinacea and aloe vera are just a few of the many complementary supplements that mix well with GSE.

What is Grapefruit Seed Extract?

Grapefruit seed extract (GSE) is a potent, broad spectrum antimicrobial that is made from the seeds, pulp and often the white membrane of grapefruit. The extract was first made only using the seeds, but then researchers realized that many properties of the seeds existed in the pulp and membranes as well.

When making the extract, the pulp and seeds are dried and ground into a powder, and then distilled in water to remove the fiber and pectin. The remaining substance is dried again into a bioflavonoid grapefruit concentrate and added to a food grade acid mixture. The mixture contains polyphenolic compounds (quercitin, helperidin, campherol, glycoside, etc.), and although polyphenols are unstable by themselves, they are converted into a stable class of quaternary ammonium compounds.

Some quaternary ammonium compounds consist of industrial antimicrobial chemicals that are toxic to humans and animals, but the nontoxic B vitamin choline—essential for some neurological and metabolic functions—is also a quaternary ammonium compound. GSE seems to have inherited the best of both worlds—it is a powerful antimicrobial without the toxic side effects of its chemically-derived relatives. It is nontoxic and derived from natural sources, as well as being tested and found completely safe, even at levels above the recommended amount. However, it is acidic, powerful and very bitter. Therefore, it is recommended that the extract be diluted a great deal, depending on usage.

Why do grapefruit seeds have such strong antimicrobial properties? Much of this answer can be traced back to the purpose of seeds in preserving plant species. Fruit trees in particular have developed elaborate ways to protect their seeds in order to ensure species continuation. Citrus fruits, in particular, have tough skins of a strong chemical make-up to protect their seeds from microbe invaders. Once the skin is compromised, the flesh itself offers little resistance for the invaders, and seeds are soft and fairly vulnerable.

So why is it that grapefruit can take months longer to decompose compared to, say, an apple? The pulp and membranes of citrus fruits contain many biochemicals dangerous to the microbes, which helps. And if the microbes make it to the seeds, with its precious genetic codes, the polyphenolic compounds in the seeds are an incredible barrier to the parasitic invaders. In fact, citrus fruits are usually unsuitable for composting, because they can take two years to decay. And so, while many seeds are toxic to humans, citrus seeds—grapefruit included—can be converted so they retain their powerful parasite-fighting properties without producing side effects.

Research history of GSE

Initiated by Jacob Harish, who studied nuclear physics in both Germany and Long Island, GSE development took a long time to flower. In fact, it wasn't until 1963, after his move to Florida, that he received the necessary funding to pursue his research on the seeds. Harish then approached two leading doctors in the field of microbes and food to push his idea. They were won over by Harish's research, and with these two doctors and the food science lab at the University of Florida behind him, other laboratories and institutions began following suit.

However, it wasn't until 1990 that Harish's discovery received the scientific credibility it deserved. And by 1995, Harish was invited out to the Pasteur Institute in France to take part in some of the leading AIDS research in Europe. There, researchers looked at the possibility of using GSE to fight secondary infections often associated with AIDS, as well as tapping into its antiviral power. In fact, since 1974 countless research labs and universities have continued to research GSE's properties and safe usage.

How does GSE work?

Currently, researchers know more about what GSE can do and safe dosages of the extract, than they do about how exactly GSE works. This is often the case, however, with new substances, whether they be artificial medicines or natural supplements. Researchers in Korea, however, are closer to the answer. From their observations, they believe that the way GSE interacts with microbes alters their cell membrane and inhibits enzymatic activity.

Other issues are still not well understood. For instance, many researchers remain baffled as to why GSE can have an effect on such a wide range of parasites without any toxicity toward humans and animals—in fact, many researchers say that a person would have to take 4,000 times the recommended amount to risk even a fifty percent chance of toxic side effects. Another issue is GSE's antiviral activity. Since viruses have no membrane, the findings in Korea do not explain GSE's effect on such viruses as influenza, herpes and measles.

Results of a GSE study at the Southern Research Institute

The results of this 1994 study named the following in a list of pathogens that GSE is effective against. GSE was twice as effective than leading disinfectants for the following:

> *Staphylococcus aureus*
> *Streptococcus pyrogenes*
> *Streptococcus fecalis*
> *Streptococcus pneumonia*
> *Klebsiella pheumonia*
> *Proteus vulgaris*
> *Pseudomonas aeruginosa*
> *Salmonella choleraesuis*
> *Escherichia coli*
> *Candida albicans*
> *Trichophyton mentagrophytes*
> *Herpes simplex virus type 1*
> *Influenza virus type A2*

GSE's antibiotic properties

THE ANTIBIOTIC DEBATE

The development of drug-resistant bacterial strains has been the subject of many magazine articles, newspaper headlines and programs recently. One type of bacteria to hit news media is the "flesh-eating bacteria", a strain of *Staphylococcus aureus,* that has claimed many lives in Europe and the United States. Many attribute the appearance of these super bacteria to doctors writing more antibiotic prescriptions than they should, and people asking for and/or using more antibiotics than necessary. In fact, it is estimated that the typical three-year-old will have had ten courses and 200 doses of antibiotics from birth. And the average person can expect to have had around 1,000 doses of antibiotics by the time they reach fifty.

Some of the other drawbacks of traditional antibiotics include toxicity, suppressed immune system and destruction of friendly bacteria in the body. Traditional antibiotics can often have side effects, cause extreme reactions, upset the digestive tract and even lead to liver damage or worse. In addition to this problem, they work by suppressing the action of the immune system and interfere with the body's natural formation of antibodies against the germ, so the chance of relapse is greater. These interferences can depress future action of organs related to immune function, as well as weakening the bodies resistance to future infection. Similarly, by interfering with the balance of natural flora in the body, candida infections can begin, which eventually lead to an overall collapse in health.

What would an ideal antibiotic be like, then? It should be powerful and effective, but not weaken the immune system. Instead, it would work with the body as a broad spectrum substance that would fight many different mixes of germs and viruses. It would be reasonably priced and derived from natural sources.

Grapefruit seed extract fits this description and is now being acknowledged and prescribed by many health care professions, as well as being used in hospitals. Not only do many hospitals disinfect their laundry and rooms with cleaning substances that contain GSE, they are also beginning, as one hospital in California has, to use GSE in respirators for bronchial infections among other things.

GSE AND THE VRE SCARE

Dr. David G. Williams, in his book *Alternatives for the Health Conscious Individual,* writes about GSE: "I find more and more uses for it [GSE] every day . . . it may be the only thing that will save your life. I've discussed how overuse and misuse of antibiotics are causing more strains of bacteria to mutate and become antibiotic-resistant. The situation continues to worsen and is far more serious than the general public has been told."

Dr. Williams then makes reference to the growing problem with a certain strain of bacteria called VREs, or Vancomycin-resistant Enterococci. This is a strain that has never received much attention, because until recently, it could be eliminated very easily with the drug vancomycin. This drug is important, because it is the last remaining treatment for life-threatening staph and strep infections.

Recently, however, starting with New York City hospital and spreading to many more hospitals, reports started surfacing about patients treated with vancomycin without success. These new strains (VREs) were not responding to the antibiotic. Even more disturbing was the fact that ninety-eight percent of them had acquired the VRE *after* admission to the hospital.

In the next few years, the Centers for Disease Control reported an increase of twenty-times the original number of cases. Soon there were reports of similar problems in France, Britain, Spain, Belgium, Sweden, Australia and many other countries. A surgical journal in Europe reported in 1994 that VREs were the most rapidly growing resistant bacteria reported by hospitals, and VREs became the second leading cause of infection developing after admission into the hospital.

VRE bacteria can survive for a week on a counter top, a day on a telephone and half an hour on the diaphragm of a stethoscope. In fact, it takes a full thirty seconds of washing with soap to get it off of the hands, and infections of VRE are practically untreatable, even with combinations of antibiotics. They occur predominantly in older people with depressed immune systems or those in intensive care, and if the infection spreads to the blood, reports the Albert Einstein College of Medicine, the death rate is one hundred percent.

However, one treatment has proven successful against this super infection—GSE. Some doctors tried a version of the extract when patients requested natural remedies to fight the infection. GSE proved to be effective in treating the infection for those patients.

GSE AND SORE/STREP THROAT

If GSE can be effective against supermicrobes, it can also help with minor infections, including those associated with sore and strep throat. Doctors doing research on the antibiotic properties of GSE say that simply gargling with water containing a few drops of GSE can handle the most resistant Strep infections, and it is not toxic to swallow. In fact, for children, diluting a drop or two of GSE into a heavy syrup is also effective and covers the bitter taste of the extract. Depending on the severity of the infection, a sufferer may see results in as little as two to three days.

GSE AND GINGIVITIS

Gingivitis is often the result of bacteria causing a plaque-build-up in the mouth that leads to swelling, redness, infection and eventually tooth loss. Sometimes vitamin deficiencies, fungi or certain viruses can cause gum disease as well. GSE diluted in water and used as a rinse can help not only with gum disease, but also mouth ulcers and general dental cleanliness. It is not recommended, however, to apply the acidic extract directly to the teeth or infected gum, as it could cause damage to the tooth enamel.

GSE AND SKIN PROBLEMS

GSE can also be effective against various skin problems or diseases either caused by a bacteria or those which could lead to a bacterial infection. Some of these skin problems include acne, dermatitis, impetigo, shave itch, cracked lips and even basic cuts and wounds. Because GSE has the power to both kill bacterial infection and disinfect to prevent infection, its topical use for skin infections is vast but effective. It can even be used (in diluted form of course) to prevent infections that arise from certain bug bites and even poison ivy and oak. In fact, GSE can be diluted with water or a calendula tincture in a spray bottle and used as a deodorant to control body odor (also associated with bacteria).

GSE'S OTHER ANTIBACTERIAL APPLICATIONS

• Sinusitis (GSE and saline solution for nasal spray.)
• Earaches (Do not use extract directly in ear; dilute.)
• Eye infections (The safety of this treatment, however, is still under debate. Do not try with children.)

HOW GSE CAN HELP FIGHT INFECTIONS ASSOCIATED WITH AIDS

Although the Pasteur Institute of France is working on a possible AIDS treatment using grapefruit seed extract, studies are still preliminary. Researchers do know that GSE has antiviral properties, but the extent of its effectiveness is still unknown; however, many AIDS or HIV patients are reporting that GSE is helpful in fending off secondary infections that often arise as the immune system weakens. Defending the body from secondary infections is the difference between life and death for many advanced AIDS patients, and is important in early stages of the disease as well. Diluted GSE mixtures should be taken internally as a preventative, topically to infections (including skin and candida infections) and can be used to disinfect food, dishes and living space, as well as in hand soaps and related items.

GSE AND OTHER SECONDARY INFECTIONS

Grapefruit seed extract can also be helpful in preventing and treating secondary infections associated with **chronic fatigue syndrome** (due to weakened immune system), **diabetes** (especially in feet, may prevent amputation) and **Lyme disease** (studies are still under way to see if GSE fights the disease-causing bacteria itself, but patients reported symptoms lessened while using the extract).

Treatment should consist of taking a diluted form internally as treatment and preventative, as well as topical uses. It can also be used to disinfect food, clean counter spaces and related areas.

GSE AS A PREVENTATIVE FOR SERIOUS DISEASES WHERE BACTERIA IS A FACTOR

Researchers are now discovering that some serious health issues, such as arthritis, heart attacks, kidney stones and ulcers, may have a root in bacterial infection, at least in some cases. GSE, then, may be useful in fending off those bacteria that can lead to more serious health problems.

Arthritis. Some forms of arthritis—especially rheumatoid—have been linked to bacterial strep for quite some time, but scientists have just begun to find connections between arthritis and two bacteria that reside in the digestive tract—*Proteus vulgaris* and *Klebsiella pneumonia*. *Klebsiella pneumonia* usually occurs in the spinal column, while *Proteus vulgaris* can cause inflammation in any joint and can lead to rheumatoid symptoms.

How do the bacteria cause the autoimmune deficiencies that lead to arthritis? Researchers believe that the antibodies that are sent to combat these antigens are absorbed by the intestines and enter the blood stream. Normally, these antibodies can then be filtered by the liver and related organs, but in some people this just isn't the case. Instead, the body starts attacking itself.

The antibiotic properties of grapefruit seed extract seem very promising in helping with this crippling disease. GSE can also help with candida and dysentery, which scientists have found can also improve symptoms in arthritis patients who had these problems.

Heart Attacks. Similarly, researchers in Britain have discovered that men who have suffered one heart attack and have antibodies for the common bacteria *Chlamydia pneumoniae* were four times more likely to have another heart attack, and that treating them for the bacteria lowered their chances of a repeat attack. Since this report, many researchers have found that lifestyle and genetics may not be the only factors that increase heart attack risk. Bacterial infection may be another one.

Dr. Sandeep Gupta at ST. George's Hospital Medical School in London said that there is a connection between antibodies and heart disease, and that this type of chlamydia bacteria, which causes a chest infection, has also turned up in plaques in the arteries of patients.

GSE's antibacterial properties may prove useful in heart disease and heart attack prevention as well. GSE may also be helpful with stroke treatment and prevention.

Kidney Stones. A recent study in Finland reported that a certain nanobacteria may be the starting point for kidney stones. They can be found in blood serum and kidney stones, and their shells are made of apatite, a mineral found in teeth and bones. When they settle, they quickly form a thick shell that scientists speculate may be the starting point of kidney stones, forming layer by layer like a pearl. They found evidence that the crystallized center of tested kidney stones was made of biogenic apatite. Because of GSE's broad antibacterial ability, it has been recommended for kidney stone prevention as well.

Ulcers. Scientists have discovered that their previous approach to ulcers may be wrong. Bacteria may actually be a primary cause behind ulcers. *Helicobacter pylori*, a bacteria that causes ulcers in pigs, has been found in twenty-five percent of humans, and it is present in more than fifty percent of those suffering from stomach and duodenal ulcers. Now it is becoming standard procedure to check for the presence of this bacteria in the sufferer.

GSE can be helpful, but it should be used with care because of the acidic nature of the extract. Start with small doses and work up, and if you experience any burning decrease your dose. Ulcers can be dangerous, so always involve a health care professional in your treatment decisions and progress. GSE may also be a good preventative.

GSE's antifungal properties

THE CANDIDA CRISIS

Candida albicans is a fungal yeast infestation that starts in the digestive and urogenital tracts, but can spread to any part of the body. Although the pathogen itself is only mildly irritating, it has the capacity to grow at a very fast rate, and once there is a yeast imbalance, even the healthiest of people will suffer the effects of it. Candida infections can show up in digestive imbalances, as well as thrush and yeast infections.

The presence of the fungus in the human body is not peculiar—most humans have at least a small amount of it in their body, but in Western societies these infections are growing out of control. Some doctors actually consider it one of the biggest challenges to good health in industrialized nations.

Candida toxins circulate in the bloodstream and cause illness. Symptoms are often varied and can often be mistaken for something else. It can produce false estrogen and make the body think it has enough and signal the body to cease production. It also can send out messages to the thyroid making it think it has enough, therefore stopping thyroxine production. These results can cause menstrual irregularities and hypothyroid problems. It can also cause fatigue, indigestion, flatulence, diarrhea, depression, anxiety, depressed libido, carbohydrate cravings, bladder, vaginal and ear infections, and skin infections like eczema and acne, as well as sometimes causing menstrual problems.

Diet, lifestyle, some prescription drugs and oral contraceptives are thought to upset the yeast balance in the body, as well as stress, sleep disorders and pregnancy. Chlorine in the drinking water also tends to upset the normal bacterial flora of the intestine. Even meat and poultry contain antibiotics that can lead to an infection.

CANDIDA AND GSE

Candida albicans can occur in both men and women. When candida outnumbers the friendly flora in the body, it quickly proliferates in the body, spreads to the blood stream and invades other tissues. It can lead to or be the result of long-term immune dysfunction and is common in AIDS patients and those suffering from chronic fatigue syndrome. To make matters worse, antibiotics only make the problem worse in most cases, especially when they are overused.

Grapefruit seed extract, however, can be very promising in helping people with candida. Dr. Leo Galland from New York, who has treated many people suffering from chronic Candida found only two failures among 297 cases. A study done at a university in Mexico tested women with vaginal infections using GSE as a treatment. Three-fourths of the women needed only one treatment, four received two before achieving results and only one patient needed three treatments.

Physicians in many hospitals and in their own practices have followed suit, since most candida treatments are highly toxic and GSE is so safe, inexpensive and often more effective. It also does not pose much of a threat to the friendly flora in the body and can actually help these good bacteria become balanced again.

A one-week cleansing diet is recommended before starting treatment, however. The following is an example of such a diet:

• Sixty-five percent high fiber, low starch raw vegetables
• Twenty percent vegetable proteins like tofu, nuts and seeds

- Ten percent complex carbohydrates like rice, beans and millet
- Five percent fruit—grapefruit, papaya, pineapple, berries

There has to be a colon and blood cleansing, and along with GSE, the body can rid itself of many toxins, not just candida. GSE should be taken between meals, unless it irritates the stomach too much. Doses are to be increased gradually over a one month period, though some people may not need to, depending on the severity of the infection. A good rule of thumb is to increase the number of times in a day you take GSE rather than immediately increasing dosage.

For vaginal infections, use GSE to make a douche. For thrush, topical and internal treatment is recommended. Use GSE as a gargle before swallowing, or use GSE to make a syrup.

RINGWORM AND GRAPEFRUIT SEED EXTRACT
Actually not a worm, this fungus of the genuses Trichophytum, Microsporum or Epiodermophytum forms a ringlike lesion that can appear anywhere on the skin. It can be the result of metabolic weakness and poor hygiene, as well as many other reasons, but can be treated with GSE very simply. GSE should be made into a spray with water or goldenseal tincture and applied to the infected area as often as necessary.

GSE'S OTHER ANTIFUNGAL APPLICATIONS
- Athlete's foot (Apply topically; wash socks in GSE solution.)
- Dandruff (Add five drops of GSE to shampoo and shake well with each wash; let stand three to five minutes.)
- Jock itch (Add GSE to body powder and apply topically.)
- Diaper rash (Apply topically, one part GSE, one part slippery elm and fifteen parts finally milled rice or corn.)
- Nail fungus (Mix one-half ounce GSE to five ounces of alcohol or vodka, apply on or under nails with eyedropper two or three times a day.)

GSE's antiviral properties

FIGHTING COLDS AND FLU WITH GSE

Several different viruses can cause what we call the "common cold" or versions of the flu. Many of these are resistant to treatments, or they mutate so quickly, that no treatment can be made to treat them without being immediately obsolete. However, GSE used in combination with other bug-fighters (including olive leaf, echinacea, goldenseal and astragalus) can be very effective against these viruses. GSE can also help with intestinal flu by attacking the parasites directly in the digestive tract. The Southern Research Institute found that GSE is particularly valuable when fighting the influenza-A virus.

At the first sign of cold or flu, take a few drops of GSE in juice or water two to three times a day, or add more drops to a quart or more of juice and sip it throughout the day. Tinctures of other bug-fighting herbs can also be used in combination with GSE. Of course, the best way to avoid a cold or the flu is prevention. GSE can fight off the germs, viruses, parasites and worms that invade the body before they become a threat if taken on a regular basis.

COLD SORES, WARTS AND GSE

Both cold sores and warts are caused by viruses. Cold sores are caused by the Herpes simplex 1 virus and usually appear on the face and lips, but they can appear elsewhere. Warts are usually caused by the activation of virus that has either just been introduced to the body or has been dormant in the body. The virus uses its own genetic information to create its own foreign tissue, and this can occur on various skin surfaces.

The Herpes virus that causes cold sores is thought by some to be found in most humans and activated in some by stress—whether it be physical, emotional or a stress to diet. GSE's antiviral and antiseptic properties seem to be able to dry up the cold sore and inactivate the virus in a couple of days and sometimes in just hours.

GSE is effective against warts because of its acidic and antiviral properties. However, warts on the genitals or near the eyes should not be treated with GSE. Some warts, including pedunculate warts, are easier to treat than plantar warts because of the location of the root.

Warts can be treated with GSE at full strength, although very carefully. Remember to use a swab to apply treatment and cover the wart with a bandage during treatment. For cold sores, however, GSE should be diluted in vegetable glycerine and applied with a swab. If you experience any irritation, lower the amount of GSE used in dilution.

OTHER VIRUSES THAT CAN BE TREATED WITH GSE

• Measles
• Animal Viruses (According to the United States Department of Agriculture, GSE was effective against foot and mouth disease, African swine fever, swine vesicular disease and avian influenza.)

How GSE can help with gastrointestinal problems

LEAKY GUT SYNDROME

Leaky gut syndrome is one condition that can lead to and may be associated with other serious disorders. The gastrointestinal tract is designed to perform many important and essential functions for the body. It digests and assimilates nutrients for use in the body. Vitamins and minerals attach to proteins to cross the gut lining and enter the bloodstream. The gastrointestinal tract also works to detoxify chemicals and harmful substances that enter the body and fight infection. If the lining of the intestinal tract becomes more permeable than normal, it can lead to serious health concerns.

The large spaces that develop between the cells of the gut wall allow toxic material to enter the bloodstream. Under normal conditions these toxic substances would be eliminated, but when leaky gut syndrome occurs, parasites, bacteria, fungi, toxins, fats and other foreign matter enter the bloodstream. These microbes can put an enormous strain on the liver and lessen its ability to detoxify, and foreign matter allowed into the gut wall stimulate immune response.

When these antibodies are produced, the body begins to recognize relatively common foods or other substances as detrimental and this leads to allergic reactions, joint problems and gastrointestinal difficulties, such as Crohn's disease or colitis. Other associated problems include migraines, eczema and immune problems. And since it lowers the immune system, it can cause frequent colds, infections, nausea and diarrhea or even fatigue.

Leaky gut syndrome is a common health condition primarily due to today's lifestyle, but many times the problem is overlooked by medical professionals. The symptoms may be masked for a time but the underlying cause remains. Poor diet, sugars, antibiotics, alcohol and caffeine can all irritate the lining of the stomach and intestines which can lead to the syndrome.

Prevention, of course is the best method. Using GSE on a regular basis can help eliminate irritating parasites, bacteria, fungi and other microbes from the intestinal walls. GSE can also help release the strain put on the immune system. However, GSE can also be used to help treat the problem, but remember that GSE is acidic and can irritate an already tender bowel lining—use at lower concentrations.

The risk of leaky bowel leads us to an even greater risk associated with a weakened immune system.

The Cancer Connection. Although we know that several factors are involved in the development of cancer, we also know that cancer is a dysfunction of the immune system. When the immune system is weakened, the body is vulnerable to abnormal cells that arise there, but if the immune system is healthy, they are detected and eliminated from the body.

A toxic body allows parasites, worms, viruses, bacteria and germs to multiply. Many doctors feel that parasites are involved with cancer. Which comes first, the parasites or the cancer? In the book *Guess What Came to Dinner*, author Anne Louise Gittleman says of parasites: "They destroy cells in the body faster than cells can be regenerated, thereby creating an imbalance that results in ulceration, perforation, or anemia. They produce toxic substances that are harmful to the body. . .The presence of parasites depresses immune system functioning while activating the immune response. This can eventually lead to immune system exhaustion."

Since the 1940s, Dr. Livingston-Wheeler and numerous other scientists have confirmed the existence of a cancer microorganism. In *Alternative Medicine Definitive Guide to Cancer* we read: "In the

1940s, the late Virginia Livingston, M.D., discovered a bacterium which she called Progenitor cryptocides . . . Dr. Livingston discovered that the bacterium caused cancer in experimental animal studies and she found it in virtually all human and animal cancers."

The risk of cancer should make us even more aware of how important prevention and early treatment of immune-weakening problems like leaky bowel syndrome are, because they lead to more serious and even life-threatening risks. Many people have been reported to have taken GSE every day for several years, without side effects. GSE is the ideal preventative to stop parasite takeover without compromising the immune system or the natural balance in the body.

TRAVELER'S DIARRHEA AND GSE

Traveling abroad has always carried the risk of diarrhea, unless you were willing to boil or chlorinate everything that came in contact with your mouth—even your toothbrush. Now, however, GSE may be the preventative you need to avoid tummy troubles associated with traveling. Some doctors even report both preventative and curative effects.

In fact, Dr. C. W. Lynn of Florida reports that he has prescribed two drops of GSE twice a day to patients suffering from traveler's diarrhea in South America with great success. Some patients even recovered within one or two days.

On another occasion, Dr. Lynn traveled to Mexico and South America with thirty-eight patients, both males and females of all ages. He had half the group take one drop of GSE in water daily as a preventative and the other half did not. No one taking GSE had any problems with diarrhea during the trip unlike many of the travelers in the group not taking GSE.

Dr. Louis Parish, MD also warns of protozoan danger: "The mobile and international society of the late 20th century has taken people to areas where they cannot avoid dangerous food." In his prospectus for the FDA, he estimates that one fifth of the world's population suffers from protozoan infections. He claims that in many parts of the world, these infections are a way of life—much like having a cold. He also warns that tourist infection is not limited to tropical areas; in fact, one in four tourists visiting Lenningrad is infected.

Dr. Parish, working as an investigator for the Department of Health and Human Services, researched GSE and found it to be "as effective as any other amoebicide now available, perhaps even more effective [because] it does not cause side effects." He treated patients suffering from both Entamoeba histolytica and *Giardia lamblia*, and he found that GSE offered more relief to patient symptoms than any other treatment.

FOOD POISONING AND GSE

The antimicrobial power of GSE is also important, considering the many problems that have surfaced around imported fruits and vegetables. Problems like cyclospora infections, among others, are causing stomach problems in a growing number of Americans. Americans do not even have to leave the country to experience the effects of microbes on food. In the spring of 1996 and 1997 in the United States and Canada, an outbreak of cyclosporiasis was associated with the consumption of fresh Guatemalan raspberries, which affected more than 1,000 individuals.

Parasites are found in the water we drink, the food we eat, and the air we breathe. The Giardia cyst can thrive up to three months in cool or cold water, and the Cryptosporidum cyst can survive for up to 18 months. Giardia is found in lakes and streams in the United States. Imported food from out of the country, may not be properly tested. Food from other countries may expose the population of the United States to *Toxoplasma gondii*, a latent parasitic infection.

Parasites are linked with other diseases such as AIDS, autoimmune diseases, Crohn's disease, and even in pulmonary conditions. Dr. Hulda Clarke, author of, *The Cure For All Diseases* believes that the most dangerous of the parasites is *Fasciolopsis buski*. These intestinal flukes live among water plants, such as water chestnuts, bamboo shoots, watercress and lotus root plants and enter the body when they are ingested.

GSE can be an effective preventative and treatment for mild food poisoning and has been used over longer periods to treat parasitic dysentery. Higher dosages can be used for dysentery, taken in juice up to every four hours over a few weeks or even a month or more. Supplementing treatment with acidophilus is also a good idea.

Food poisoning may also be avoided by washing foods in water mixed with a few drops of GSE to kill microbes—even Salmonella. In fact, new drug resistant strains of Salmonella have been reported recently by the head of the Central Public Health Laboratory in London. Infections by these strains are on the rise, and these infections are resistant to nearly one hundred percent of available antibiotics.

Raw meat, fruits and vegetables in particular should be washed with a GSE mixture before preparation. In fact, counters, dishes, cutting boards, pans and knives should also be disinfected using GSE, because it is effective and nontoxic. GSE can even be added to your washer to disinfect kitchen towels—GSE is more effective than chlorine bleach and safer. It is also more cost effective.

GSE'S OTHER GASTROINTESTINAL USES
• Nausea
• Stomach flu
• Flatulence

Note: GSE can also be used as a colonic.

Other uses for GSE

GSE FOR ALLERGIES
Allergies are a disorder of the immune system. The colon and digestive system plays an important role in the prevention of allergies. Irritations from environmental, food and air pollutants can cause a weakening of the mucous membranes in the body, making them permeable and allowing toxins to enter the bloodstream. Food and toxins that make contact with weakened digestive tract can cause irritations and sensitivities.

When food is eaten and digested, it enters the bloodstream, the body recognizes them as nutrients and utilizes them. When undigested food enters the bloodstream, the body considers them as foreign invaders and attacks them as if they were bacteria or viruses. GSE, however, can encourage proper immune function, thereby discouraging these digestive problems and the resulting allergies. It does so by clearing the gastrointestinal tract of unwanted guests, so that immune response can be redirected towards fighting allergens in the forms of toxins and related items.

THE ANTIOXIDANT PROTECTION OF GSE

Free radical damage is the result of unstable molecules that cause many health related ailments. Free radicals are not all bad, and in low doses, they are useful in helping to kill bacteria. However, when antioxidants and oxygen are lacking in the brain, damage results. If the free radicals attack DNA, it could cause birth defects. If the pancreas is damaged, it could develop into diabetes; cardiovascular diseases can occur if the blood and blood vessels are damaged. If the eyes or ears are damaged, it could cause cataracts or hearing loss. Free radical damage has also been linked to senility and related problems.

We know that oils become rancid quickly when oxidized. Scientists call the process of fats turning rancid, lipid peroxidation. Oxidation can occur in our food such as wheat, grains, oils, nuts, seeds and many prepared food on the grocery shelves. It is also caused by air pollution, cigarette smoke, environmental chemicals, radiation and heavy metal poisoning.

GSE can be an excellent antioxidant and can prevent these problems. GSE contains tocopherols, citric acid and ascorbic acid, and a study done at the Universidad Pedagogica Experimental Libertador in Venezuela showed the antioxidant effects of GSE on vegetable oils. It was discovered that GSE at high temperatures actually has a prooxidant effect, but at low and normal temperatures, it does exhibit antioxidant properties. Researchers concluded that GSE could not be used in oils used for cooking and frying, because the high temperatures would block their antioxidant effects; however, fats and oils stored at room temperature for an extended period of time could benefit from GSE.

In addition, the *Journal of Agriculture and Food Chemistry* also supports claims about the presence of antioxidant activity in grapefruit juice and pulp.

GSE LIMONOIDS FOR CANCER AND CHOLESTEROL

What are Limonoids? Limonoids, recently popular in many scientific circles, are bitter bioactive compounds found in large quantities in citrus fruits, including grapefruit. They are now being studied predominantly for their anticarcinogenic properties. They have also been shown to possible help with cholesterol management. They are easily extracted from the peel, the seeds and pulp. Limonoids are also a natural extract and carry many benefits that artificial drugs do not. They are found in only two plant families—citrus and mahogany—and act as natural plant-protecting agents.

Limonoids and Cancer. Compounds in limonoids have been tested on human tissue and proven effective against mouth, throat, lung, stomach, colon, skin, liver and breast cancers. The University of Minnesota discovered that the cancer-fighting chemicals in limonoids stimulate enzyme production in the liver, producing GST (glutathion S-transferase). This enzyme has the ability to detoxify carcinogens. Many types of limonoids produce this effect, particularly nomilin and limonin. Studies done by Felicia So. Najla Guthrie and co-workers at the University of Western Ontaia, Canada, indicated that limonoids and limonoid glucosides can have a beneficial antitumor effect. The studies in animals show these compounds are metabolized after oral ingestion. This implies that the normal consumption of citrus fruits, coupled with GSE supplementation, could offer significant anticancer help in humans.

Results on humans are preliminary, but it seems to be very promising and without side effects. Studies are continuing.

Limonoids and Cholesterol. The limonoids, which are concentrated in the grapefruit seeds and pulp, show promise in reducing low-density cholesterol in rabbits. The early implications of these findings show that these compounds can help in eliminating or reducing plaque from the artery walls.

LDL cholesterol ("bad" cholesterol) is the type which can cause serious damage to the artery walls. It contains a chemical known as apolipoprotein-B, which is responsible for the problem. The apolipoprotein-B adheres to arterial walls, resulting in plaque build-up, and inhibits the smooth flow of blood. When the adherence is near the heart, the individual is at risk of developing coronary heart disease. High LDL cholesterol levels have been linked to heart disease, which can lead to a heart attack or stroke. HDL cholesterol is thought to be the "good" cholesterol. It is considered to be beneficial in protecting the arteries. It may actually prevent the cholesterol from adhering to arterial walls. High HDL levels are helpful in preventing heart disease.

Grapefruit seeds contain oils made up of six fatty acids, both saturated and unsaturated—myristic, palmitic, stearic, oleic, linoleic and linolenic. These and the limonoids in GSE could be responsible for its cholesterol-lowering effects.

HOUSEHOLD AND GARDEN USES FOR GSE
- KEEP humidifiers mildew free.
- CLEAN fish tanks of algae.
- ALTERNATIVE to chlorinating pools and jacuzzis.
- DISINFECT laundry safely.
- CLEAN kitchen surfaces, play areas and bathrooms.
- WASH dishes, utensils and pots and pans.
- USE as a fungicide/viricide instead of pesticides on home gardens.
- USE to treat water when camping or in emergencies.
- MIX with cleansing and soap products for bodily and house use.
- STERILIZE areas to prevent the spread of infection or illness.
- SANITIZE razors, toothbrushes and other hygiene items.
- CLEAN shower mildew.
- USE to wash raw meats, vegetables and fruits before preparation.
- PREVENT microbe infection on household plants and flowers.
- ALTERNATIVE for waste water treatment.
- USE for well-cleaning.
- DISINFECT doorknobs, tile, garbage cans, pet and child areas, keyboards, toys and telephones.
- ADD to patching and caulking to prevent mold and mildew formation.
- USE in primer and finish coats in painting, stains, sealers and finishes, especially in areas where humidity is high or where paints will come in contact with water (like bathrooms), to prevent mildew and fungi.
- USE in cleaning products at nursing homes, day-care centers, etc.

- ADD to rug cleaner and/or steamer to kill bacteria, mold, spores, fungi and parasites.
- ADD to water kept in storage—cisterns, cooling towers, etc.

PETS AND GSE

Household pets and farm animals can also benefit from the powerful nontoxic antimicrobial GSE. Whether they suffer from skin diseases, injuries, fungal infections or any diseases caused by bacteria, viral, fungal or other microbes, GSE can help.

GSE is a broad-spectrum fighter, making it ideal for animals, who can't tell us what is wrong. It can be mixed with food or topical sprays, shampoos, flea dips—even litter and bedding. Once again, the rule of thumb for internal use is to increase the times a day GSE is administered, rather than the dose itself. GSE always needs to be diluted. Child dosages are good for small animals.

GSE can be both a treatment and preventative. It will not harm your animal to administer a small dose daily. It has been determined to boost immune systems in animals and lower mortality rates. Veterinarians reported particular success with problems like gas colic, rashes, cat flu and minor injuries.

Dosage and Safety

GSE dosage varies, depending on the potency of the GSE extract you are using; however, GSE in almost all cases, should be diluted since it is very powerful. Stronger concentrations can be used for disinfecting and cleaning surfaces, laundry, etc. Dosages for children and small animals should usually be at least half the size of adult dosages. In general, increase the times a day you take GSE before bumping up the dosage amount too much. It can be used both internally and externally. It can be diluted in water, juice or syrups for ingestion and in shampoos, lotions, oils, water, alcohol, etc. for external use.

GSE is safe to take as a daily preventative in small amounts. Sometimes treatment can be as little as one or two days, but for more serious problems, treatment should go on for a few weeks or even a month. Do not apply concentrated on the skin, except in the event of a blister or related skin problems.

A NOTE CONCERNING SAFETY

Recently, reports have surfaced about GSE containing preservative chemicals, including triclosan, benzelthonium chloride and methyl paraben. In particular, studies from Japan and Germany, including a study from a 1999 issue of *Pharmazie*. These studies claim that GSE holds not antimicrobial power of its own, but rather gets its power from these chemical preservatives and that these preservatives are not safe.

However, GSE has a makeup very similar to some of these dangerous chemicals—toxic to humans. However, the GSE testing for these chemicals actually produces a "false positive," meaning that because of the similarity between the safe agent GSE and the harmful chemicals, tests came up with an inaccurate positive for the chemicals. Many GSE-producing companies have since ran tests for these chemicals that have come back negative. **GSE is effective, nontoxic and very safe.**

THE HERXHEIMER EFFECT

Another thing to keep in mind when taking GSE is the Herxheimer or "die-off" effect. Although there are no side effects associated with GSE, when it is used to treat a chronic condition there may be an adverse reaction by the body. This reaction is not to be interpreted negatively, however. It is actually a sign that the body is recovering from illness.

This effect is basically the result of GSE's effect on the invading microbes in your body. As GSE is implemented, the body with the help of the immune system will begin a process of removing toxins from the body. If there are large numbers of these microbes, the body may develop symptoms like headaches, swelling of the mouth, throat, sinuses or lymphatics, rashes, fatigue, diarrhea, muscle aches, joint pain or other flu-like symptoms.

The "die-off" effect is not singular to GSE, but is actually common with any microbe-killing agent or with any substance used to detoxify and cleanse the body. However, despite the seeming adverse effects of antimicrobics like GSE, these symptoms are actually a sign that the body is healing, and that it will feel a whole lot better after die-off.

Drinking plenty of water can minimize die-off effect. Temporarily reducing the GSE intake can also reduce symptoms. However, the die-off effect is generally not long-lived, depending on the degree of microbe infestation.

Complementary supplements to use with GSE

Aloe vera. This herb can be used both topically and internally for its soothing powers and mild cleansing activity.

Astragalus. A Chinese medicinal used in the treatment of cold and flu, as well as immune boosting.

Echinacea. This is one of the most well-known herbs for immune defense. It can be taken with GSE at the onset of infection.

Garlic. Often used for the immune system in Chinese medicine, ayurvedic medicine and now in the American mainstream. It has both antiviral and antibiotic qualities.

Goldenseal. It was used by Native Americans to treat infections, because of its alkaloidal effect on bacteria and viruses.

Licorice. A popular herbal used to fight bacterial and viral infections and stimulate the immune system.

Mushrooms. Many Asian mushrooms (including cordyceps, shiitake and maitake) are known for their immune-boosting abilities.

Noni. A powerful all-around antimicrobial that has been used to treat various degrees and types of infections and immune deficiencies, as well as a number of diseases.

Olive Leaf. This extract is a potent antimicrobial that fights bacterial and viral infections.

Pau d'arco. This herb has powerful antiviral, antibiotic and immune boosting abilities.

Peppermint. Not only soothing, this mint and others also show antiviral properties. Cloves and cinnamon also are antimicrobial.

Tea tree oil. A powerful topical antimicrobial.

Vitamin C. One of the top vitamins to fight cold and flu, and build the immune system.

Zinc. Zinc has been known to fight colds, and a zinc deficiency has been linked to immune disorders. Zinc lozenges are recommended.

Bibliography

Armando, Carrasquero, Salazar Maythe and Navas Petra Beatriz. "Antioxidant Activity of Grapefruit Seed Extract on Vegetable Oils." *J Sci Food Agri* 77(1988), 463-67.

Bennett, Raymond D. "Acidic Limonoids of Grapefruit Seeds." *Phytochemistry* 10(1971), 3065-68.

Bennett, Raymond D., Shin Hasengawa and Zareb Herman. "Glucosides of Acidic Limonoids in Citrus." *Phytochemistry*. 28:10(1989), 2777-2781.

"Citrus compounds have anti-cancer, cholesterol-lowering effects, say researchers." *Food Labeling News*. April 7, 1999.

Crowell, Pamela L. "Prevention and Therapy of Cancer by Dietary Monoterpenes." *Symposium on Phytochemicals: Biochemistry and Physiology*. 1999.

Elkins, Rita. *Hawaiian Noni*. Lindon, UT: Woodland Publishing, 1998.

The GSE Report, 1:1 (1999), 1-15.

Gould, Michael N., PhD. "Prevention and Treatment of Mammary Cancer by Monoterpenes." *Journal of Cellular Biochemistry, Supplement*. 22(1995), 139-44.

Hasegawa, Shin, Raymond D. Bennett, Zareb Herman, Chi H. Fong and Peter Ou. "Limonoid Glucosides in Citrus." *Phytochemistry*. 28:6(1989), 1717-20.

Hawken, C.M. *Natural Cold and Flu Defense*. Lindon, UT: Woodland Publishing, 1997.

Manners, Gary D. and Shin Hasegawa. "Squeezing More from Citrus Fruits." *Chemistry and Industry*. 19 July 1999, 542-46.

Nutriteam. "Grapefruit Seed Extract". http://www.nutriteam. com/gsewhat.html, http://www.nutriteam.com/3opinion.htm, accessed 11/15/99.

Parasites, Parasitic Diseases and your Health. Com/parasites. htm.

Parasites, The Hidden Health Threat, What Doctors Don't Tell You. July 1999.

Ritchason, Jack. *Olive Leaf Extract*. Lindon, UT: Woodland Publishing, 1999.

Sharamon, Shalila and Bodo J. Baginski. *The Healing Power of Grapefruit Seed*.

So, Felicia V., Najla Guthrie, Ann F. Chambers, Madeleine Moussa and Kenneth K. Carroll. "Inhibition of Human Breast Cancer Cell Proliferation and Delay of Mammary Tumorigenesis by Flavonoids and Citrus Juices." *Nutrition and Cancer*. 26:2(1996), 167-81.

Sachs, Allan D.C., C.C.N. *The Authoratative Guide to Grapefruit Seed Extract: A Breakthrough in Alternative Treatment for Colds, Infections, Candida, Allergies, Herpes, and Many Other Ailments*. California: Life Rhythm, 1997.

Teles, F.F. Feitosa. Triglyceride Fatty Acids of Arizona Grapefruit Seed Oil. *Journal of Food Science*. 37(1972), 331-2.

Tenney, Louise. *The Natural Guide to Colon Health*. Lindon, UT: Woodland Publishing, 1997. 87-94.

Uedo, Noriya, Masaharu Tatsuta, Hiroyasu Iishi, Miyako Baba, Noriko Sakai, Hiroyuki Yano and Toru Otani. Inhibition by D-limonene of gastric carcinogenesis induced by N-methyl-N'-nitro-N-nitrosoguanidine in Wistar rats. *Cancer Letters* 137(1999), 131-6.

Wang, H., Cao, G, Prior, R.L. Total antioxidant capacity of fruits. *Journal of Agriculture and Food Chemistry*, 4:3(1996), 701-5.

Woedtke, Th. Von, B. Schluter, P. Pflegel, U. Lindequist and W.D. Julich. Aspects of the antimicrobial efficacy of grapefruit seed extract and its relation to preservative substances contained. *Pharmazie* 54:6(1999), 452-56.